Cover : Apple Blossom at the Living Proof by Ann Peckham

Some interior photos: Michelle Payne-Gale (MPG), Essence Photography

Disclaimer: The information contained in this booklet is not intended as medical advice. Ann Peckham does not recommend cooked foods or standard medical practices. The author, publisher and/or distributors will not assume responsibility for any adverse consequences resulting from adopting the lifestyle described herein.

The Uncook Book Taster : a gradual introduction into the very easy creation of nutritious and delicious alternatives to the usual suspects

Copyright © 2011 by Ann Peckham; Publisher: lulu.com

ISBN-978-1-4477-7804-2

This booklet is dedicated to all of my students and customers who have waited so patiently for the publication of "The Uncook Book for the Busy and the Lazy"

This is to get you started on the road of recovery in the simplest and most convenient ways possible.

And a huge thank you to my mother, Mrs I Peckham, for supporting me and believing in me, without her help this book would have taken a lot longer to get to print.

With lots of love and light

Ann

Contents

Introduction

I have always found that there is far too much padding in self-help books so there are pages to plough through before you get to the nitty gritty. This book will get you straight into what you really want to have a go at and that is making really easy foods that are good for you.

Everything in here can be made with minimal ingredients and equipment you are likely to already own, even if it is kept hidden in a cupboard. Most of them can be made in less than 15 minutes. All of them taste great and better than that they can help your mind and body improve on many levels.

At the end of the book you will find some useful information that will help you to make wiser choices if improving your health levels is your aim.

The first section on Green Smoothies is enough to get you started on the right track and they have the potential to help you feel so much better that your cravings for less healthy options will start to diminish and you will want to include some of the other foods in your diet too.

This book could very well start you on the road that will lead you to more energy, stronger immune system and an improved zest for life. I really hope that you will enjoy experimenting with these recipes and gain the confidence that will enable you to create your own versions as do my students.

So without further ado let us proceed.

Green Smoothies

One of the most health promoting and important groups of foods that is virtually completely missing from our diets and is completely missing from the "Food Pyramid" is green leaves and the healthiest way to eat them is raw. The very thought of ploughing through plates piled high with kale or spinach and chewing them until they form a liquid in our mouths before we swallow (as our stomachs don't have teeth) is enough to make you cringe and worse than that, not do it at all.

Greens make the body more alkaline (which we need to do if we want to regain our health) and contain the super healing powers of chlorophyll. Since ancient times chlorophyll has served as a miraculous healer. Some of the healing properties are;

- Builds a high blood count; counteracts toxins eaten; helps purify the liver; helps sores heal faster; eliminates body odour; improves varicose veins; reduces pain caused by inflammation; soothes painful haemorrhoids and piles; helps prevent cancer and improves anaemic conditions.

I got turned on to green smoothies through the work of Victoria Boutenko www.rawfamily.com reading her book "Green for Life" ISBN 0-9704819-6-9 in it you can read testimonies about how green smoothies have transformed the lives of ordinary junk food eating American folk (and they are the champions at that). There is the story of an experiment carried out for 30 days with group of people from a small town called Roseburg in Oregon. They tell of weight loss, increased energy, better sleeping patterns, depression lifted, less blood sugar fluctuations, more regular bowel movements, asthma attacks stopping completely and an inner glow.

A body that has access to the most powerful nutrients on the planet no longer craves food because it has been given what it needs to renew itself.

When you habitually feed it foods that are virtually devoid of nutrients then your body will set up powerful cravings in an attempt to make you eat the foods that it needs for its self-healing system to function effectively. But if you keep feeding it dead, toxic foods you will never quell the cravings and so you end up in a vicious circle which seems impossible to break out of. Because of this automatic mechanism it really isn't your lack of will power that is preventing you from losing weight or regaining your health it is the consequence of the choices you make given the information you have.

Making green smoothies

There are just three main elements to these and if you vary them and mix and match you will find that you have a huge variety;

- the choice of greens; the choice of fruit and the liquid

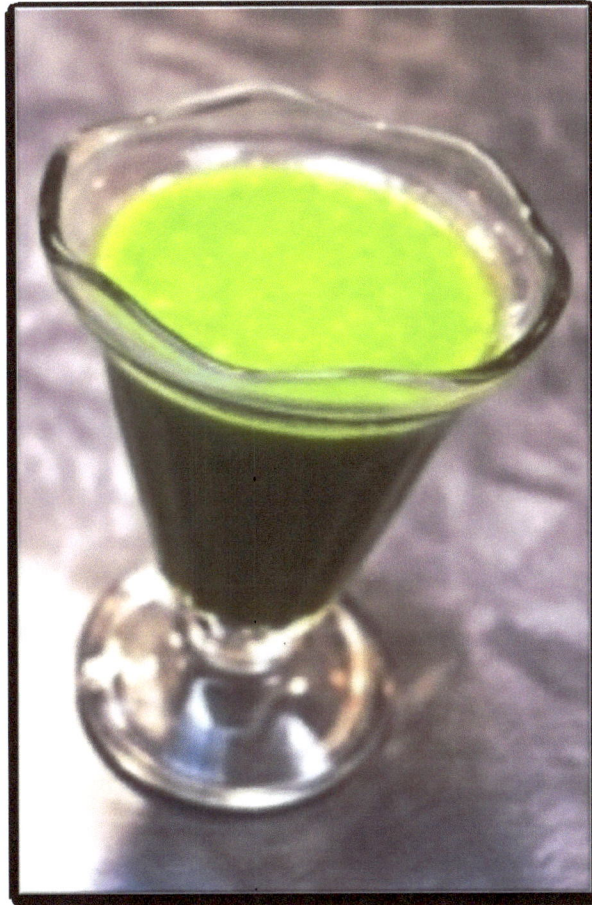

Greens;   Figure 1 Green Smoothie

- Spinach; kale; spring greens; young dandelion leaves (they aren't bitter) ; romaine lettuce; bok choy, carrot tops (the green leaves that grow out of the top of the carrot or any other root vegetable), rocket and so on.
    - o Do try to get organic greens wherever possible so that you take in the minimum amount of toxins.

o Remove the heaviest stalks (they can make it a little bitter) and rip into pieces to make the blending easier.

o It is advisable to rotate your greens because eating the same greens every day can cause problems in the long term.

o This really is a great area to experiment with because you will discover that each green tastes different.

o When you get adept at making green smoothies you will find that you become much more adventurous and will develop an interest in gathering wild greens which are even more nutritious than shop bought ones and they are free too. If you look at the end of this booklet you will find a list of edible greens including "weeds".

Fruit;

- Banana; mango; papaya; blueberries; strawberries; peaches; goji berries; black cherries; raspberries, red/black currants and so on, have fun and experiment.
    o Do make sure that the fruit you use is ripe and preferably organic
    o Chop it up to make it easier for the blender and remove any stones

Liquid;

You can use filtered water which makes perfectly acceptable drinks and I find that using a shop bought juice can really help to improve the flavour and if the main aim of this green smoothy is to ingest more greens easily then the better it tastes the more likely you are to make them a regular habit.

Make sure that you select the best quality juice at the price you can afford. If you can find freshly squeezed variety they won't have pasteurized it, the enzymes will still be intact which is better for you.

- Apple juice; Apple and Mango; Apple and Pear; Pineapple and Passion Fruit; Passion fruit Pear and Apple; Freshly squeezed Orange juice and so on
    o Each juice makes the smoothy taste different so it is entirely up to you which variety you use dependant on your taste buds.
    o If you have a juicer then you can freshly make your own liquid and really have fun, though this will take up a lot more of your time as you will need to clean it out immediately for ease.

- Carrot, apple, celery and cucumber are a good mix and are great on their own as well as mixed into a green smoothy

Method

This couldn't be simpler;

- peel the fruit (if it needs peeling) chop it up and put it into the blender first
- Add a little of the juice and blend till liquid
- Add 1 or 2 large handfuls of green leaves, any hard stalks removed.
- Add the rest of the juice and blend till all of the leaves are broken down and the smoothy looks smooth
- Pour into a glass and drink slowly, chewing it to mix it with saliva (an important part of the digestive system)

So once you have found a selection of ingredients you like the taste of and you have got into the habit if doing this most if not every morning then you will be able to use the smoothy as a carrier for other super foods which will really help to boost your immune system.

NB. *Because digestion starts in the mouth it is very important to "chew" your smoothy, this may seem weird but if you get your food to start breaking down in your mouth it removes the need for your stomach to have teeth! Remember also that the mouth contains saliva which is an important part of the digestion process.*

Some additional healthy additive suggestions

A ripe avocado; cashew nuts; coconut water or milk; Aloe Vera Gel; Spirulina.

- Avocado and the cashew nuts will give the smoothy a rich thickness, you can get these anywhere
- The raw cashews that you can buy in town are theoretically not completely raw because heat is used to extract them from their shells however the certified 100% raw variety are very expensive so as long as the ones you buy are not roasted and salted you should be ok.
- Coconut water and milk; contain no appreciable levels of cholesterol. They increase the speed of the thyroid allowing the body to lose weight and toxins. Coconut oil cannot be

stored in the body as fat, it need to be burned on the spot, which fires up our excessive fat burning metabolism.

- Aloe Vera; is great for your body - both internally and externally. Aloe Vera has some fantastic natural healing benefits which is why it has earned the title "miracle plant"
- Spirulina: contains high concentrations of 18 vitamins and minerals; rich in chlorophyll. Contains all essential amino acids; 65% of Spirulina is protein; rich in gamma-linoleic acid (GLA) - an anti-inflammatory Omega 6 fatty acid; rich in phytonutrients and antioxidants

So experiment and have fun and start the journey back to health the easy way!

Your feedback please.

It would be really valuable to hear if you notice any difference from drinking green smoothies so please take a note of how you feel and what ailments you have before you start and then again a month later and then email me the results I would be very interested purpleann57@yahoo.co.uk

Questions to ask yourself before you commence, there are no right or wrong answers (make sure you write the answers down as memory can let us down!)

1. What is your standard diet prior to commencing green smoothies? (what foods and drinks to you habitually consume)
2. What health issues do you have? (both physical and mental)
3. If you are overweight, by how much and for how long have you been trying to lose weight?
4. What are your sleeping patterns?
5. What are your elimination patterns?
6. What are your energy levels?

Questions to ask yourself after a month of green smoothies

1. How easy did you find drinking up to a quart of green smoothy per day?
2. Did the rest of your diet change at all as a result of the green smoothy, if so in what ways?
3. Did you notice any changes in your health, if so what were they?
4. Did your cravings for unhealthy foods lessen?
5. Did you notice any change in your weight?
6. Was there any change in your sleep patterns?
7. Did your energy levels change, what did you notice?
8. Did you have any symptoms of detox, if so what were they?
9. Did you have any negative experiences?
10. Will you continue to make and drink green smoothies?

Risotto; (serves 4 as a starter or 2 for a main meal)*

You will need a food processor to make this but you can do it in a small one a little at a time

Ingredients

- A medium organic cauliflower
- A red or orange pepper
- 4-6 spring onions
- 3-4 Tbs Flax oil
- 1 tsp turmeric
- 2 tsp cumin
- 1 tsp ground cardamom
- ½ tsp Himalayan salt

Method

- De seed and finely chop the pepper; I use a small "dicer" to get evenly sized pieces
- Finely slice the spring onions all of the white and a little of the green.
- Pour the flax oil into a small bowl and add the spices mix well.
- Break the cauliflower into small flourettes remove all of the leaves and the larger stalky bits. Place in the food processor with the "S" blade and break down into rice sized bits.
- Place cauliflower into a large bowl and add all of the other ingredients, mix together well so that everything is evenly spread throughout. It will have a slightly yellowish tint to it because of the turmeric, this will show you that you have mixed it well because if you haven't there will still be white bits
- Transfer to flattish dish and spread risotto evenly, cover with a lid.
- Place in oven on at the lowest setting at the bottom with the door slightly ajar for an hour or so
- You can also warm this through by placing it in a bowl and putting that bowl into a slightly larger one that has hot water

in it. Cover with a plate to keep the heat in and stir it every 5 minutes or so to warm through evenly.

- Eat it whilst it is still warm otherwise it can be safely eaten the following day if you simply transfer it into a container after it has cooled down. Because this risotto isn't made with rice it is safe from the toxins you get from cooked rice.

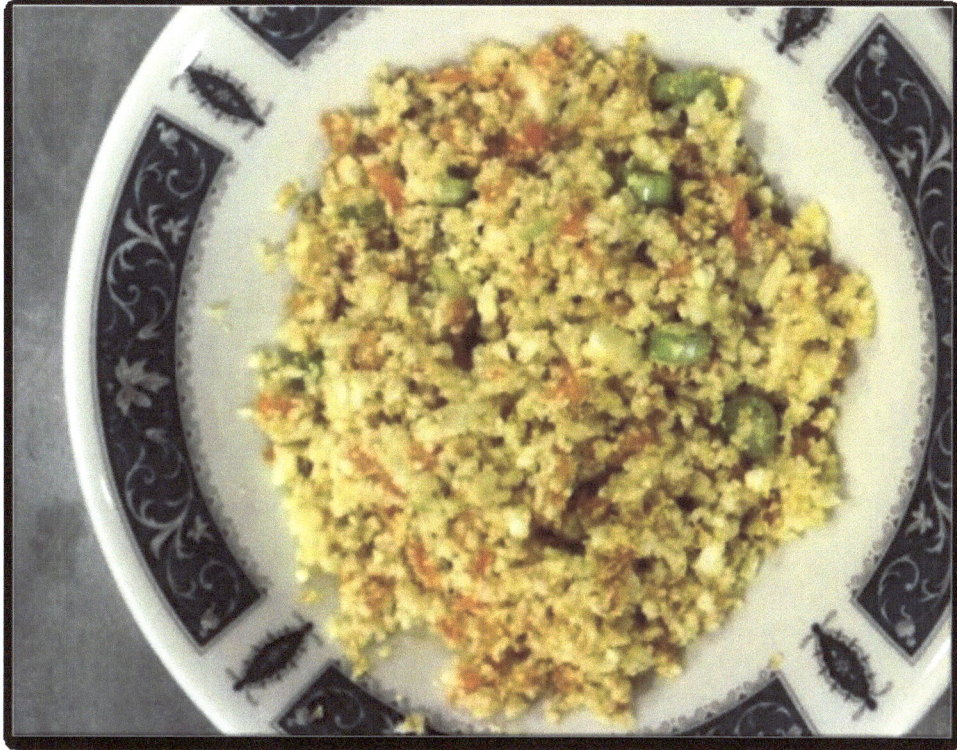

Picture 2 Risotto

- I have been making this meal for years and cannot recall who inspired me with its creation. Whoever did I am eternally grateful as this is so simple and so tasty.

Mushroom Quiche Creamy version

(makes 1 large for 4 or 4 small individual ones)

Base Ingredients

- 2 cups Almonds
- 1 cup rolled oats
- 1 Tbs Tahini
- 1 Tbs Dark Miso
- 4-6 Tbs water

Method

- Break down the almonds in a food processor until they look like fine bread crumbs
- Add the oats to the food processor on top of the almonds and mix till they are flour like, you are still likely to have little bits of almond which is fine
- Mix the tahini, miso and water together,
- Put the almond mix into a bowl and pour the tahini mixture over it mixing thoroughly
- Press into a flan dish using the back of a dessert spoon, lining the base and sides with a crust about ½ inch thick. Put to one side in the fridge. You can also make individual ones for lunch boxes

Filling ingredients

- 2Tbs Tamari
- 2 Tbs Olive oil
- 1 cup cashews
- 2 Tbs Nutritional yeast
- Clove garlic
- 1 Tbs Psyillium husks
- 8 Mushrooms
- ¼ cup filtered water

Method

- Finely slice the mushrooms with a mandolin (this is really fast and you get even slices) and place in bowl.
- Mix together the Tamari and olive oil and pour over sliced mushrooms coating well, leave to marinate for an hour or so
- Put the cashews into the blender with the nutritional yeast, garlic and water and blend till smooth
- Add the Psyllium husks and blend again briefly as these will thicken the mixture.
- Transfer the mixture to a bowl, drain the marinate from the mushrooms and add them mixing carefully not to break them up too much
- Spoon the sauce into the base, and smooth over

Leave for an hour or two in the fridge to set and serve with a green salad. Will keep for 4-5 days in the fridge and easily freezes. This is so delicious that you will want to make a batch and keep in your freezer for a quick and nutritious meal.

Picture 3 Mushroom Flan with Green salad

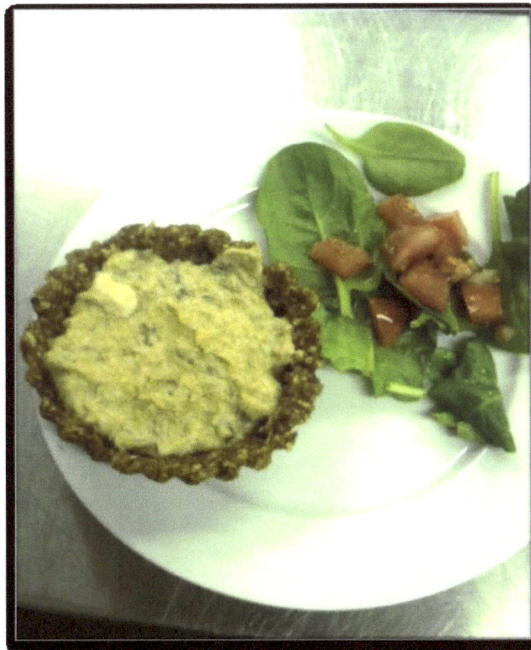

Brilliant Beetroot Soup.

Ingredients: (serves 2-3)

- 2 raw beetroots topped, tailed, peeled and quartered
- 1 sweet apple, cored and quartered
- 1 medium tomato, quartered
- 1 carrot, peeled and sliced
- 2 Medjool dates, de-stoned
- 1 desert spoon of agave nectar (optional)
- 1 Tbs of Flax oil (or hemp or olive) and Tamari
- 2 Tbs of nutritional yeast flakes
- 300-400ml filtered water boiled then allowed to cool a little
- 1 handful of Pine nuts

Method

- Place the tomato, dates, agave nectar, oil and Tamari into the blender and blend till smooth
- Add the apple, Nutritional Yeast flakes and the beetroot and add the warmed water half at a time (this is so you can get the thickness you prefer)
- Blend till as smooth as you can make it,

Serve immediately sprinkled with pine nuts, enjoy!

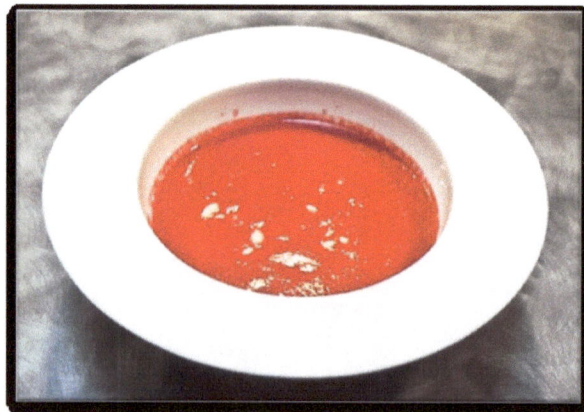

Picture 4 Brilliant Beetroot Soup

Tropical Soup

(Inspired by Karen Jessett from "Clear Skin" www.acne-advice.com)

Ingredients (Serves 3-4)

- 2 mangoes
- 2 passion-fruit
- 2 Tbs fresh ginger, grated
- ½ red onion finely chopped
- ½ avocado finely chopped
- 2 tomatoes deseeded and finely chopped
- 300ml fresh orange juice
- ½ red bell pepper, finely chopped
- Handful of fresh coriander finely chopped
- Juice and zest of lime

Method

- Peel and chop the mangoes into small pieces and place in bowl
- Spoon out the seeds and flesh of the passion-fruit and add to the mangoes with the ginger
- Marinate in the fridge for 30 minutes
- Blend the mangoes and marinade with the orange juice
- Mix the onion, tomato ,avocado and bell pepper in a bowl to make a salsa
- Pour the mango liquid into individual bowls and mix in lime juice then top with the salsa
- Finish off with chopped coriander and lime zest and serve

This is such an easy soup to make and it is so delicious both sweet and savoury. Served cold it is fabulous in a hot day and really impresses people.

The original recipe uses chilli peppers but I found that far too hot!

Pecan Nut Pate

Ingredients

- 2 cups Pecans soaked
- 1 cup leeks finely chopped
- 2 Tbs olive oil
- 1 Tbs Italian seasoning
- ½ tsp Himalayan salt

Method

- Process all with the "S" blade of the food processor adding a little water for consistency
- Store in a sealed container in the fridge

This is so easy to make you will realise how simple it is to eat more healthily

Picture 5 Pecan Nut Pate

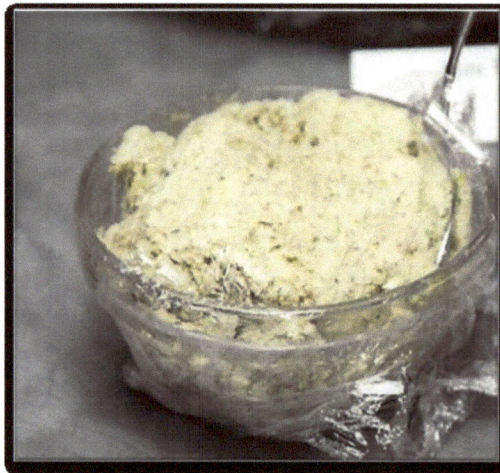

Tomato Salsa Serves 2-4

Ingredients

- 4 Plum Tomatoes
- A handful of fresh coriander
- 1 clove garlic finely chopped
- 2 Tbs chives finely chopped
- 2Tbs fresh lemon juice
- ¼-½ tsp cayenne (to taste)
- Himalayan salt, to taste

Method

- Cut the tomatoes into quarters and remove the seeds and the tough green bit
- Finely cube the tomatoes,
- Holding the fresh coriander by the stalks on the chopping board remove the stalks. Keeping the leaves together chop them finely, you will find that after chopping for a little while you will be able to hold the knife at both ends thus keeping your fingers out of the way of the blade
- Place the tomatoes and the chopped coriander into a bowl and mix in all of the other ingredients
- Transfer to a sealed container and store in the fridge
- This tastes great immediately and will improve over the next couple of days
- Can be kept for 1 to 2 weeks in a fridge

Picture 6 Tomato Salsa and Mexican Crackers

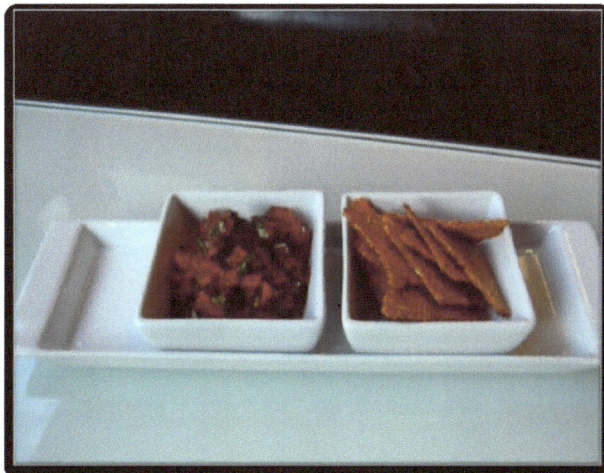

Tomato and Chilli Relish*

Ingredients (serves up to 4)

- 2 Tomatoes
- 2 sun dried tomatoes chopped
- ½ small onion chopped
- ¼ red hot chilli de-seeded and chopped
- A handful of basil leaves
- 3 soaked dates
- 1 clove of garlic
- 1 Tbs Tamari

Method

- Place the fresh tomatoes with the Tamari, dates and garlic into the blender and blend till liquid
- Add the sun dried tomatoes, onion, chilli and basil leaves and continue to blend till desired consistency
- Serve with salad and raw crackers or as a relish with anything else you eat
- If you find that the final result is too runny, adding a couple more sun dried tomatoes with thicken it up spectacularly
- Do remember to use dried tomatoes, not roasted or stored in oil!

* I was inspired to create this recipe by Jess Fenton www.totalrawfood.com back in 2007 when I attended a training day in the Earth Ship near Brighton; thank you we all love this recipe!

Caesar Salad (Serves 3-4 as a side dish)*

Ingredients

For the salad

- ½ head Chinese leaves
- ½ cucumber
- ½ red pepper
- ¼ cup of red onion
- 1 large carrot
- ¼ cup desiccated unsweetened coconut

Method

- With a sharp chef's knife cut straight across the Chinese leaves 1/4 " thick and place in large bowl
- Peel and slice the cucumber into ¼" thick slices then chop into cubes
- Chop the red pepper into small cubes
- Chop the onion and grate the carrot
- Add everything to the bowl and mix thoroughly

For the dressing

- 2 Tbs olive oil
- 1 lemon juiced
- 1Tbs honey
- ½ tsp cumin powder
- 1 large clove garlic crushed
- ½ tsp Himalayan salt

Method

- Place the ingredients in a container with a screw lid and shake thoroughly till well blended
- Pour over the vegetables and mix well before serving

* I was inspired to create this salad by experimenting with a recipe I found in "A Complete Book of Raw Food" the original of this was accredited to Jalissa Letendre. I love the flexibility of raw foods it really inspires creativity.

Purple Ann's crunchy salad

Ingredients; for the salad (serves 2)

- 3 cups of Baby leaf spinach
- 1 cup coriander (cilantro), finely chopped removing the large stems as these can be rather wood like
- 4 Tomatoes, quartered, deseeded and cubed
- ½ cup red cabbage finely grated
- ½ cup sunflower seed sprouts or un-sprouted
- 1 Avocado diced
- 1 carrot grated
- ¼ cup red onion finely chopped
- 10 black olives finely chopped
- 1 Tbs hemp seed shelled

Method

- Place all of the ingredients into a large mixing bowl and mix well

Ingredients; for the dressing

- ¼ cup lemon juice
- 1 Tbs honey
- 1 Tbs Tahini
- 2 Tbs Braggs liquid aminos

Method

- Place in a screw topped container and shake well and pour over salad, and enjoy

Picture 7 Purple Ann's Crunchy Salad Variation

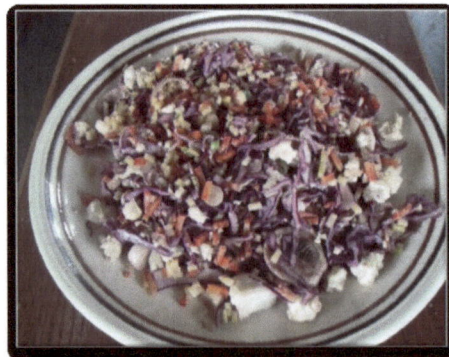

Apple Pie

(Makes a large pie that will easily serve 8)

Ingredients; Base

- 200g of Almonds **not** soaked
- 100g fresh and dried dates about 50g of each
- Coconut butter to bind 50g melted (by standing a small bowl of coconut oil in another larger bowl which has hot water in it, this will turn it from a soft white solid to a clear liquid)

Topping Ingredients

- 2 Apples ¼ and cored
- 110g Fresh dates cut up small
- 1 desert spoon of mixed spice
- 1 lemon freshly squeezed
- 1 large orange peeled and de-pipped
- 1 inch peeled ginger or ½ tsp dried ginger
- Handful of raisins
- 2 tsp Psyillium husks

Method

Base

- Add the almonds to the food processor almonds to break them down before you add the dates and blend till it resembles small bread crumbs
- Add the melted coconut oil at this point and pulse till it starts to stick together
- Press into a spring form cake tin and refrigerate

Topping

- Put the dates, spice, orange, ginger and lemon juice into to the blender and blend till smooth.
- Add the apple and raisins and blend slightly so that there are still bits visible

- Add Psyillium husks and blend for about 3-4 seconds, this helps to solidify the mixture and stop it sliding off the base.
- Add the topping to the base evenly and smooth with the back of a spoon
- Leave to settle in the fridge for at least 30 minutes

This is delicious on its own and even better served with cashew nut creem*

Picture 8 Apple Pie

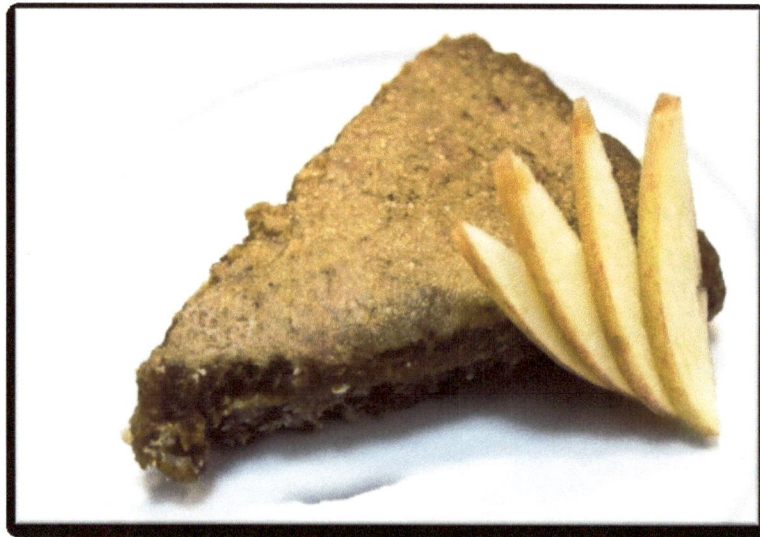

*Cashew cream

This is so simple to make and can be made very quickly you can even make it without soaking the cashew nuts

Ingredients

- 1 cup of cashew nuts soaked for 4 hours
- ½ cup of fresh dates or ¼ cup maple syrup or honey
- 1 tsp vanilla extract
- Water to desired consistency.

Method

- Add everything to the blender with a small amount of the filtered water and blend till smooth
- Add more water gradually till desired thickness achieved

Do keep in mind when you are adding the water that it is always possible to add more water but impossible to take it out if you have added too much so add it gradually.

Another thing to be aware of is that if you are using un-soaked cashews they will absorb water and the creem will get thicker if you leave it over-night. This can be stored in a sealed container in the fridge for well over a week and you can beat in more water or coconut water if it gets too thick.

Fruit Moose

These are some of the easiest and most delicious creamy desserts and they can be made very quickly.

If you have spent the past years trying to control your calorie intake you are likely to feel both deprived and resentful. This is very disheartening for the soul as it spoils the enjoyment of life.

So when you taste a fruit moose made from one of your favourite soft fruits it will tick all of the boxes for flavour and even better than that it will be really good for you.

Black Cherry Moose

Ingredients

- 1 cup of black cherries (you can use frozen ones but please defrost them by standing them in a bowl standing in hot water. This is important otherwise when the melted coconut oil comes into contact with the frozen fruit it will re-solidify)
- 1 handful of cashew nuts
- 2 Tbs honey (or maple syrup or agave nectar), both available in most food shops
- 3 Tbs coconut butter/oil melted
- 2 Tbs coconut milk (you can get this in tins, so choose the organic version)

Method

- Using the blender blend the black cherries with the honey and the coconut milk until it is smooth
- Add the cashew nuts and blend again until smooth
- Add the melted coconut butter and blend till there are no lumps at all
- Pour or spoon into serving bowls and cover with cling film and put into the fridge to set

You can make a whole range of fruit mooses by changing the fruit, I make strawberry, raspberry, summer fruit, fruits of the forest, black forest fruits (frozen from a supermarket) mango, papaya, pineapple, nectarine or any other favourite soft fruit. This is an area that you can experiment with to your heart's content and see what you come up with; let me know if you get a really good one.

5 reasons to switch from eating wheat, dairy or sugar

1. Do you remember when you were little what you used to make out of mixing flour and water together? Yes that is right it was GLUE! So it is not surprising that you feel stodged up after eating bread, nor is it any surprise that more and more people are becoming intolerant to wheat.

2. Have you ever noticed that you feel sleepy in the afternoon if you have eaten sandwiches for lunch? Wheat and other grains have a soporific effect on the body, in other words it sends you to sleep.

3. Dairy has been proven to cause a build-up of mucus in the body which clogs things up and leads to sinusitis and hay fever amongst other things.

4. Humans are the only creatures on the planet to consume the milk of another animal and we are the only ones to continue to do so after weaning.

5. Refined sugar is one of the most damaging to health leading to diabetes, raised blood pressure and heart problems. Most refined sugars are found within simple carbohydrates such as breads and pastas, or added to processed food to make them more palatable.

There is more information about this in

"Fabulous Cakes, Decadent Desserts and Heart Healthy Chocolates"

Acid and Alkali forming foods*

The human body is incredible in its ability to heal itself given the right environment. Remember as a child how quickly you recovered from any bumps and scrapes and how that is not so nowadays as the aches and pains make you feel your age.

This need not be so as the human body still has amazing recuperative abilities when you know how to achieve it. The main problem the body has with trying to recover itself is caused by having too acidic environment caused by eating acid forming foods. The most acid forming foods are as follows starting with the worst culprits.

Acid Forming Foods

- **Meat:** including fish, poultry and game.
- **Dairy:** Cheese, Eggs and milk. Remember that milk is for infant animals and not needed beyond that stage.
- **Sugar:** all kinds of sugar and all sugar-containing products such as biscuits, cakes, jams, soft drinks, ice-cream.
- **Condiments:** pickles, sauces, tea and coffee and alcohol (apple-cider vinegar is ok)
- **Grains:** Wheat, rice, oats, barley and all flours and breads. If you can soak and sprout them they are less acid forming.
- **Beans:** Soya, broad, kidney
- **Legumes:** Lentils, chickpeas, peanuts and peanut butter
- **Nuts:** Walnuts, cashews, pecans, if these are soaked then they are much more alkali.
- **Seeds:** sunflower, pumpkin and sesame seeds all of these are less acidic when soaked and sprouted.

If you aim for about 20 per cent of your diet to be made up of acid forming foods that will enable your body to rebalance itself and regain its capacity to heal. If you assume that the items at the bottom of this list represent a much lower percentage of the total than those at the top it makes it easy to work out which are beneficial for you to eat and which are potentially damaging and you could consider cutting from your diet.

Keep in mind that acidity in the body leads to toxicity and then on to disease.

There are some of our foods that could be regarded as neutral and that don't tip the balance either way these are;

Neutral Foods

- **Garlic.**
- Some seeds such as quinoa (pronounced keenwa)
- **Fats:** Flax, hemp, olive, sunflower, sesame, safflower.

If you aim to make up 80 per cent of your diet from Alkali forming foods then you will give your body the best chance of healing itself and finding its own natural balance.

Alkali forming foods in no particular ranking

Fruits: Apples, apricots, bananas, cherries, currants, dates, figs, gooseberries, grapefruit, grapes, kiwis, lemons, limes, oranges, mangoes, melons, nectarines, papayas, peaches, pears, pineapples, raisins, raspberries, strawberries. All of these as long as they are ripe because if they are not ripe they will be acid forming.

Nuts and seeds: Almonds, brazils, chestnuts, hazelnuts, pine kernels/ seeds used as grains such as millet

Vegetables: Asparagus, aubergines (eggplant), avocadoes, beans (runner and French) beetroot, broccoli, Brussels sprouts, cabbage, calabrese, carrots, celeriac, celery, chicory, chives, courgettes (zucchini), cress, cucumber, dandelion and other weeds and herbs, endive, kale, kohlrabi, leeks, lettuce, marrow, mushrooms, mustard, onions, parsnip, peas, peppers (red, yellow and orange as the green ones are not ripe) radishes, spinach, spring onions, squashes, sweet potatoes, swedes, tomatoes, turnips and watercress

A lot of the alkali forming foods can be eaten in a raw state which leaves their minerals, vitamins and enzymes alive and therefore useable by the body. If you feel that you need to cook some of the vegetables to make them more palatable for you then lightly steaming them will be the most beneficial way of doing this. You may find though that there are some really excellent recipes that will show you new and interesting ways of preparing vegetables without exposing them to high levels of heat.

* Reproduced with the very kind permission of Elaine Bruce http://www.livingfoods.co.uk/ in Ludlow at the start of my journey.

Reduction of cholesterol

Goji Berries

Have the ability to combat oxidation of cholesterol by increasing the body's production of SOD i.e. Superoxide Dismutase

Superoxide is one such free radical implicated in the onset and progression of aging and disease, and is neutralized by the antioxidant enzyme superoxide dismutase (SOD). As we age our body's production of this important antioxidant declines, yet Goji berries have been shown to greatly increase its presence in the body.

Goji berries are one of the most nutritionally dense foods on earth and have a staggering concentration of vitamins, minerals, amino acids, phytochemicals and essential fatty acids. Originating in Tibet and greatly favoured in traditional medicine, these scarlet berries have a mild sweet flavour between that of a cherry and a cranberry. Aside their many noted health benefits (from boosting immunity, **lowering cholesterol,** and enhancing vision to fighting cancer cells, relieving depression and **aiding weight loss**) Goji berries are touted anti-aging marvels and are one Hollywood's hottest new foods.

Goji berries are one of the highest antioxidant foods on the planet, with an ORAC score (Oxygen Radical Absorbance Capacity - a measurement used by the US Department of Agriculture for total antioxidant capacity) of 18,500, way above other fruits and veggies (blueberries, for example, having 2,200 ORAC units). Antioxidants are known for their anti-aging and disease-fighting properties by subjugating the attack of hazardous free radicals in the body.

Coconuts

Contain no appreciable levels of cholesterol. They increase the speed of the thyroid allowing the body to lose weight and toxins. Coconut oil cannot be stored in the body as fat, it need to be burned on the spot, which fires up our excessive fat burning metabolism.

They support healthy cholesterol formation in the liver as high density lipoprotein (HDL) which is essential to healthy hormone production.

Coconut oil (and all saturated fats) has been blamed for many years as a cause of bad cholesterol levels, which supposedly leads to heart disease. But studies done on traditional tropical populations that consume large amounts of coconut oil show just the opposite. One of the best ways to study the effects of coconut oil on human nutrition is to look at tropical populations that get most of their caloric intake from the saturated fat of coconut oil. Logic would dictate that if the saturated fat/cholesterol theory of heart disease and obesity were correct, those populations with the highest consumption of saturated fats would be the most overweight and have the highest rates of heart disease. Such is not the case.

In a study published in 1981, the populations of two South Pacific islands were examined over a period of time starting in the 1960s, before western foods were prevalent in the diets of either culture. The study was designed to investigate the relative effects of saturated fat and dietary cholesterol in determining serum cholesterol levels. **Coconuts were practically a staple in the diets, with up to 60% of their caloric intake coming from the saturated fat of coconut oil.** The study found very healthy people who were relatively free from the modern diseases of western cultures, including obesity and heart disease. Their conclusion: "Vascular disease is uncommon in both populations and there is no evidence of the high saturated fat intake from coconuts having a harmful effect in these populations."

Benefits of adding green leaves into your diet

- We are approximately the 7th generation of people living on processed foods
- White flour, white sugar, artificial additives, and many other additives have contributed to deficiencies and toxicity
- The dramatic reduction of green leaves from our diets is possibly the most detrimental choice we have made for our health.
- Vitamin K deficiency includes
  - Skin cancer; liver cancer
  - Heavy menstrual bleeding
  - Nose bleeds
  - Haemorrhaging; easy bruising
  - Osteoporosis
  - Haematomas

Unfortunately Vitamin K is the least studied one, ALL GREEN LEAVES ARE ABUNDANT IN IT

This group of vitamins merits a closer look; our body requires vitamin K to maintain proper functioning.

Vitamin K is known to improve blood flow and regulate clotting. Clotting is often thought to be a bad thing, and while it can be devastating in certain contexts, the body needs its blood to clot or else it couldn't properly react to wounds. **Vitamin** K actually plays many roles in regulating the overall health of blood vessels. It also promotes healthy bones and the proper growth of bones.

A deficiency in vitamin K may also have serious implications for the liver and the intestines, and one of the most serious threats involves calcium being deposited into soft tissue, effectively hardening blood arteries.

Some of the richest sources of vitamin K from vegetables include chard, turnip greens, beet greens, spinach, collards, alfalfa, kale, cabbage, Brussels sprouts, and mustard greens. Certain fruits are also rich in the vitamin, such as blueberries, kiwis, grapes, and plums.

Edible Greens

Cultivated

Amaranth; Beet greens; Bok Choy; Carrot tops; Celery; Chard; Collard greens; Cucumber leaves; Endive; Kale; Mitsuna; Mustard greens; Lettuce (all types including red); Pumpkin or squash leaves; Radicchio; Radish tops; Romaine lettuce; Salad burnet; Spinach; Turnip greens; Wheatgrass

Wild and weeds

Chickweed; Clover; Dandelion (greens and flowers); Knotweed; Lambsquarters (fat hen); Lovage; Malva; Oxeye daisy flowers and leaves; Plantain; Purslane; Rose leaves and flowers; Sorrel; Stinging nettles; Watercress; Wild mustard; Wild strawberries; Yellow dock

Herbs

Baby dill; Basil; Coriander; Fennel; Lemon balm; Mint; Parsley; Rocket (arugula)

How it came about why to incorporate them

Victoria Boutenko story;
The family had been raw for more than 11 years having become so after complete despair when doctors had given up on them;

- Husband (Igor) had been ill since childhood; at 38 had progressive hypothyroidism and rheumatoid arthritis was given 2 months to live
- Daughter (Valya); asthma and allergies
- Son (Sergei) type 1 diabetes (Victoria researched and discovered the detrimental effects of insulin)
- Victoria; arrhythmia, oedema, weighed 280 pounds

Had changed to 100% raw over night to save their lives, health improved so quickly they ran, as a family, a 10 kilometre race only three and a half months later.

Then several years later started to go backwards; knew raw veganism was the best way and didn't want to give it up but knew something must be missing; researched again; studied diet of chimpanzees; found they ate large proportion of green leaves every day

Really difficult to consume large quantities as they require long and arduous chewing sessions and depleted hydrochloric acid in modern day stomachs, body will reject them because it can't digest them, so needed to find another way of consuming them. Tried blending, smelled so disgusting couldn't even taste them. Added fruit; never looked back, hence the birth of Green Smoothies!

Multiple benefits and goodness in greens

Chlorophyll

- It has been seen to help in the growth and repair of tissues.
- Helps in neutralizing the pollution that we breathe in and intake every day - a good supplement for smokers.
- It efficiently delivers magnesium and helps the blood in carrying the much needed oxygen to all cells and tissues.
- It is also found to be useful in assimilating and chelating calcium and other heavy minerals.
- It had been seen to have a good potential in stimulating red blood cells to improve oxygen supply.
- Along with other vitamins such as A, C and E, chlorophyll has been seen to help neutralize free radicals that do damage to healthy cells.
- Chlorophyll may be useful in treating calcium oxalate stone ailments.
- It possesses some anti-atherogenic activity as well.
- It has antimutagenic and anti-carcinogenic properties so that it may be helpful in protecting your body against toxins and in reducing drug side effects.

Calcium: Studies have shown that **vegetarians** absorb and retain more calcium from foods than do non-vegetarians. Vegetable greens such as spinach, kale and broccoli are good sources of calcium from plants.

Importance of rotating greens
Almost all greens in the world contain minute amounts of alkaloids. Tiny amounts can't hurt you but if you continue to consume a single

variety of green for may weeks then the same type of alkaloid can accumulate in your body. So if you regularly get into the habit of using different greens you will never run the risk of alkaloid build up and will in fact be strengthening your immune system as well as all the other benefits.

Farewell for now

There are many different opportunities to experience what living the uncooked lifestyle feels like and if you would like to be kept informed about easily accessible and reasonably priced events then please register your interest on

www.sparklingnergy.co.uk

I will be publishing a range of books on specific topics, such as

"Fantastic Cakes, Decadent Desserts and Heart Healthy Chocolates";

"How to Impress Your Non-Raw Guests";

as well as the larger more in depth

"Uncook Book for the Busy and the Lazy"

By registering on my website you will get up to the moment updates on when events are happening and when the next book will become available.

I would like to express my gratitude to all of the wonderful people who have believed in me and who have spread the word about how it is possible to turn the tide and reclaim a strong immune system that will work to bring us back into balance, you know who you are.

I would particularly like to thank;

Elaine Bruce; http://www.livingfoods.co.uk/

Jess Fenton; http://www.totalrawfood.com/coach/

Karen Knowler; http://www.therawfoodcoach.com/

Peter Pure; http://www.rawfoodparty.com/

www.ingramcontent.com/pod-product-compliance
Lightning Source LLC
Chambersburg PA
CBHW060810270326
41928CB00002B/47